Pocket Guide to

Migraines
and
Headaches

Pocket Guide to Migraines and Headaches

Dr Edmund Critchley
D.M., F.R.C.P.

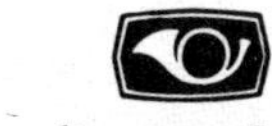

Arlington Books
King St, St James's
London

POCKET GUIDE TO MIGRAINES AND HEADACHES
First Published 1980 by
Arlington Books (Publishers) Ltd
15–17 King St, St James's
London SW1

Reprinted 1982

This revised edition first published 1988

© Edmund Critchley 1980

British Library Cataloguing in Publication Data

Critchley, Edmund
Pocket guide to migraines and headaches
— 2nd ed
1. Man. Head. Headaches   2. Man. Migraine
I. Title
616'.0472

ISBN 0-85140-744-7

Typeset by Inforum Ltd, Portsmouth
Printed and bound in Great Britain by
Richard Clay Ltd, Bungay, Suffolk

CONTENTS

Millions of healthy, normal people have headaches. Headaches vary in severity from a niggling nuisance to a pain exceeding that of cancer; and there are fortunate people who have never had even the mildest discomfort. When a headache comes, it may be totally unnoticed by one's friends and work-mates. It may be possible, even with severe pain, to continue working. Thus it is regarded as a harmless condition. If one complains about the condition, one is accused of being a misery. If one continues to complain, or has to stop work, one may be accused of malingering or of being a hypochondriac. The plight of the sufferer is poorly understood.

Between 6–10% of people are prone to chronic headaches, and these are sufficiently frequent and severe to cause loss of time from work or school. More time is lost to industry from sickness than from strikes; and headache ranks next to bronchitis and rheumatism as a potent cause of absenteeism, often afflicting those with great ability and drive. Plenty of research is being done into how headaches occur and how an acute attack can be helped. But by the time the attack has come it may be too late to treat. We must, therefore, also consider how we can alter our world by examining our mode of life, watching what we eat, drink or smoke, or by taking medicines so that we may ease the pain, or, better still, stop the headaches occurring.

An attack is a reminder of human frailty. It makes us worry. It stirs the tension within us. Often the headache sufferer has heard of a friend or relative who has had a brain tumour, suffers from epilepsy or has been psychiatrically ill, and he wonders whether he, too, is heading for disaster. He may be frightened to go to his doctor. Yet when at last he seeks medical help, has described his symptoms and been examined, he will usually accept the diagnosis of migraine, or other types of headache, with a sigh of relief. Once a diagnosis is made of the cause of the headache, the complaint can be more readily understood, he can try to recognize what brings on the symptoms, and if need be can adjust his life-style to avoid further attacks or reduce their severity in future. The aim of this booklet is to provide a guide to self-help and understanding.

DIFFERENT TYPES OF HEADACHE

A headache is not a disease. It is a complaint, a symptom. There may not always be a simple cause for a particular headache. Thus, there may be several reasons why a headache should come at a particular time. The sufferer may be depressed as he is recovering from 'flu. He may have mild sinusitis, have banged his head or received bad news. His normally brief headache may be prolonged because he is also worrying about his job. By describing many types of headache and how they can be caused I hope to give a broader idea of what a doctor will want to know about you and your headaches, and at the same time this will enable you to understand how you may help yourself avoid further headaches and deal with the problems they cause. All too often when one visits the doctor, one forgets to tell him important facts — which the doctor, God bless him, cannot be expected to know — and these facts may go far to sorting out your problem.

Most recurrent or chronic headaches are due to migraine, to tension or depression. Just occasionally other types of headache, for example those due to injury or to sinusitis, may become recurrent. Let us therefore consider a simple classification of the various types of headache.

Chronic or recurrent:
(1) Migraines
(2) Tension and muscular headaches
(3) Combined migraine and tension headache
(4) Headaches brought on by emotion, such as depression

Non-recurrent:
(5) Headaches with a vascular basis caused by:
— raised blood pressure
— anaemia
— the effect of drugs
— hormonal problems
(6) Headaches with fevers
(7) Headaches from anatomical structures
— from sinuses
— from the neck
— from the eyes
— from the ear and bones
— from the teeth and the jaw
(8) Headaches following injury
(9) Headaches with a neurological basis
— related to tumours or infections
— due to bleeding or clots
— due to arteritis in the elderly
— benign intracranial hypertension
— related to epilepsy
— neuralgic pain

Migraine

The basis of migraine is an excessive sensitivity of the blood vessels of the head. This sensitivity involves arteries and capillaries over the face and scalp and inside the skull, and occurs in attacks lasting several hours but separated by far longer periods of freedom. Why blood vessels respond in this way and to what they respond are questions which have puzzled scientists for centuries. Typically, at the beginning of the attack the blood vessels narrow down and become constricted. As a result the blood supply is reduced: not necessarily to all of the head, but parts of the brain, the eyes or the nerves are deprived of oxygen. So the attack may begin with a warning phase consisting of blurring of vision, numbness, or other sensations depending upon which part of the head is temporarily short of blood and oxygen. As the constriction wears off, the headache begins to develop, the blood vessels widen and dilate, the distended vessels stretch pain-sensitive structures through which they run, and muscles may become tense and contract.

There need not always be a clear separation between the stages when the blood vessels constrict and then dilate. The blood vessel wall may swell, reducing the flow of blood through its centre and increasing in size as it does so. Irritative substances may then seep from the blood through the wall and into neighbouring tissues. Thus it is possible to endure the discomfort of the headache and suffer from other symptoms concurrently. What is totally unexplained is why some parts of the head are involved in a particular attack but not others, and why the headache of migraine frequently involves, but not always so, one half of the head.

In migraine the disturbances can be quite complex and are not necessarily limited to the head. Thus there may be:

(1) Changes in mood with feelings of well-being just before the attacks start and later irritation, depression and even aggression.
(2) Changes in sleep and wakefulness. Before the attack one may feel sleepy and start yawning as the attack commences. Afterwards people often feel more awake.
(3) Changes in appetite. It is not unusual to feel ravenously hungry before attacks and quite unable to eat during the attack.
(4) Changes in weight. For a few hours or even days before an attack there may be increased thirst and fluid retention by the body with weight gain and ankle swelling, and during

and after the attack weight is lost again, and one may pass excessive quantities of urine.
(5) Changes in sensitivity to smells and noises which are often heightened during the attack.

Such constitutional changes explain why migraine is more than a fanciful corruption of an old French word for headache, and it is not surprising that this tendency or susceptibility to migraine is frequently inherited.

During the course of a lifetime, a person with migraine will find that the disorder may take several forms. In childhood the tendency may show as periodic vomiting. The headaches may be short-lived but violent. In later age, as the tendency slowly wears off, other complaints such as dizziness occasionally replace the more usual headache. At any age, a migraineur is just as susceptible to muzzy heads or tension headaches as other people. Migraine, alas, confers no special immunity from other disorders.

When listening to a person recount his story of migraine, a doctor is prepared to accept much variation. Not everyone's attack is identical, and some may be quite bizarre. However, he will have in his mind a list of carefully examined facts upon which to base the diagnosis. Migraine, typically, is an intermittent, often one-sided, headache with total freedom between attacks. The symptoms last from 2–30 hours and are accompanied by visual or stomach disturbances (for example, vomiting or feelings of sickness). The value of such a definition becomes clear if it is appreciated that a doctor is interested not only in diagnosis but in recognizing other factors which may, for instance, prolong the attack. Thus he might ask whether his patient has taken an excessive amount of tablets, is over-anxious, depressed, anaemic, has sinusitis, or whether there are environmental factors at his work or at home which the subject may not have recognized, or from which he cannot readily escape. Migraine most certainly can be provoked by stress. However, most migraine attacks tend to occur early in the day and — apart from cluster headaches — are the only headaches regularly causing a person to wake with pain. There are other important pointers to diagnosis:

(1) A particularly devastating headache may come after a long interval of freedom.
(2) 14% of women subject to migraine have a definite tendency to have attacks before periods (premenstrual migraine).
(3) There may be a cyclic tendency. Thus some people have their attacks when under stress

       mid-week and others as a let-down headache at weekends.

(4) Disturbances in weight, sleep, mood, appetite, etc. may be related to attacks.

(5) There may be neurological symptoms such as numbness over one side of the face, pain in the upper jaw involving the teeth, blurred or partial loss of vision.

(6) There may be, at times, weakness or numbness down one half of the body occurring on the same side as the headache.

Colour changes, palpitations (the heart racing or appearing to change gear), prominent or pulsatile vessels over the temples and forehead, are less certain features which are taken into account in making a diagnosis of migraine. In doubtful cases, as in childhood migraine, where the headpains are brief a positive history of migraine in other members of the family may help confirm the probability.

Tension headaches

Surveys of headache in general practice, or of those attending migraine clinics, include between 30–40% of headaches diagnosed as pressure or tension headaches. Possibly some unusual forms of migraine are also included, but stress in our daily lives is an important factor which we try to disregard. The basis of a tension headache is contraction and tensing of muscles over the scalp, forehead, back of the head, upper part of the neck and about the jaws. Tension headaches characteristically occur in the middle of the day, afternoon or evening. They may be brief or continue for days at a time. The severity varies: sometmes the pain will be of low intensity but persistent, boring, sharp — like a knife, bursting or exploding, or — commonly — as a feeling of a tight band around the head. The head may feel as though compressed and squeezed in a vice. Some descriptions of the headache may be colourful and melodramatic.

Analgesics relieve headpain, and tranquillisers relieve tension, but there are dangers in their continued use. To seek out the underlying cause of tension, the subject has to be considered as a whole in relation to his family and to his work. Marital disharmony, not necessarily his but perhaps involving a son or daughter, may be a source of trouble. Financial worries, mortgages, buying and selling houses, a delinquent juvenile, a shady transaction, an alcoholic spouse, an ill or demanding elderly relative, psychiatric illness in the family, fear of cancer (cancerophobia), recent deaths, operations involving relatives or even chance acquaintances, represent a string of possible sources of worry which need to be recognized and discussed. Could there have been some slight or affront, lack of compensation for an accident, a debt ignored, an imposition, underpayment for extra duties, a missed promotion, a switch to a less interesting or arduous job, or a threat of redundancy? Such factors are rarely volunteered, but a sympathetic listener can gain the confidence of the sufferer and go far to alleviate the distress. We translate many of our psychological problems into physical illness.

In the United Kingdom psycho-sexual problems do not receive as much attention as they do in the United States of America. Nevertheless, in a recent study, 50% of the patients with a diagnosis of tension headaches had psycho-sexual problems. Half the females had consulted a gynaecologist, Out of 37, 9 had hysterectomies, 1 had been raped and others had less serious but clearly defined problems. Psycho-sexual problems highlight the importance of human relationships as a cause of tension states.

We are all aware of minor problems in our lives as a cause of headache, but it is the frequency with which more serious problems thrust themselves forward in any analysis of headaches which is quite staggering. Reassurance and modification of attitudes and life-styles produce more cures than repeated prescriptions for analgesics and tranquillisers.

Combined migraine and tension

Stress is a potent cause of migraine. For a third or more migraineurs, headache is a combination of migraine and tension pains and attacks appear unduly prolonged. As Dr Oliver Sacks has written: 'Compact and clearly defined at its centre, migraine diffuses outwards until it merges with an immense surrounding field of allied phenomena.'

In the past a favourite definition of migraine has been as a headache which will only respond to ergot derivatives. This view is fallacious. At the Princess Margaret Migraine Clinic in London, it has been shown many times over that the best treatment for migraine is often a simple analgesic, such as aspirin or paracetamol, taken as soon as possible at the commencement of an attack. To prescribe simple analgesics is not to deny the diagnosis of migraine, and — by the same token — the use of a tranquilliser or an antidepressant may be equally helpful in reducing the frequency of attacks. In a recent survey, gynaecological and marital problems were recognized in a third of women with migraine and, as stress was often the culprit, the patients were advised to modify their life-styles and attitudes to avoid 'setting themselves up' for attacks.

Rudyard Kipling may well have been suffering from tension plus migraine when he wrote to Miss Margaret Burne Jones: 'Do you know what hemicrania means? A half-headache. I've been having it for a few days and it is a lovely thing. One half of my head in a mathematical line from the top of my skull to the cleft of my jaw, throbs and hammers and sizzles and bangs and swears while the other half — calm and collected — take note of the agonies next door. My disgusting doctor says it's overwork again and I'm equally certain that it rose from my suddenly and violently discarding tobacco for three days. Anyhow it hurts awfully, feels like petrification in sections and makes one write abject drivel.'

Emotionally derived headaches, including depression

'Terrible pains in the head.' 'Pain at the top of the head.' 'A numb pain over part of the head' — may bring a depressed or anxious person to the doctor. Headaches are socially acceptable, whereas ideas of self-reproach, guilt or remorse are not. When depressed, a person subconsciously may latch on to or accentuate minor symptoms such as backache, tension headache, palpitations, breathlessness or diarrhoea. Migraine rarely begins after forty and depression, arthritis of the neck, hardening of the arteries or blood pressure troubles represent more likely alternatives in the older person who has not been previously subject to migraine. Depression is an important diagnosis. It always requires early medical attention and even the more serious forms are accessible to modern treatment.

There are two kinds of depression — reactive and endogenous (inborn). Reactive depression comes with stress, such as with bereavement, particularly if the person felt emotionally 'bottled up' at the time. It may follow illness caused by viruses, for example influenza or hepatitis. Endogenous depression arises from within and may be less readily recognised. The manic-depressive personality has swing-like fluctuations of mood. In the manic phase he will be active and expansive, and during the depressive phase will lose weight, become inactive, depressed and withdrawn. An active person may lose interest on retirement or at the menopause due to an involutional melancholia. Self-poisoning from drugs or from alcoholism may also lead to depression. The consumption of these commodities by the population as a whole is horrendous and cannot be ignored. Depression following childbirth is rare but may give rise to alarm. Like other forms of depression, it is amen-

able to prompt treatment. Premenstrual depression occurring before periods is well recognized,
but seldom severe. Even so your doctor can do
much to help.

One of the features of depression may be a
variation in mood throughout the day. Sleep disturbances, such as early wakening and failure to
return to sleep, should bring the diagnosis to
mind. For no apparent reason the intake of fluid
may become excessive with the continuous im-
bibing of cups of tea or coffee, bottles of spirits,
sherry or cider, or even compulsive water drinking. Poor appetite and weight loss are common-
place but the fact may be hidden by false claims of
dieting. There may be loss of sexual drive (libido),
evidence of difficulty in arranging one's thoughts,
poor memory, a morbid outlook, feelings of self-
reproach or remorse, and these feelings may
eventually take on a delusional or hallucinatory
quality. The lesson is never to trifle with depression. Always see your doctor.

Vascular headaches

Vascular headaches can arise from changes in the
blood supply to the head. If there is an excess of
red blood cells (as in polycythaemia), the blood
will be stickier and its flow reduced. If there are

too few cells (as in anaemia), less oxygen will be carried to the brain. Loss of blood may reduce the amount reaching the head. One cause may be internal bleeding into the gut and this may produce sensations of faintness and the passing of black, tarry, bowel motions. Hormonal changes, due either to an excessive production of hormones by the glands or the use of large doses of specific hormonal drugs, which may be necessary in treating certain diseases, can result in headache, but this fact is unlikely to be of major concern. More worrying can be 'cough headache', — headaches due to repeated coughing as may happen with someone ill from bronchitis — which can result from a temporary increase in pressure within the head. If these headpains are persistent, treatment will be required from your doctor; but it is unwise, without consultation, to use large quantities of cough suppressants.

The question of raised blood pressure and headache often worries lay people. Does high blood pressure (hypertension) cause throbbing or bursting headache? It can, but only in exceptional circumstances is this the first symptom of the disease. More usually, those with mild increases in blood pressure, often an indication in itself of anxiety, are prone to tension headaches and these may be treated as such.

Fear of headache from neurological procedures, such as lumbar puncture, is very much a thing of the past due to changes in the technique and the needles presently in use. Such headache is now a rare, trivial and readily treatable complaint which need never be a source of worry.

Vascular headaches due to medicines and drugs

The proverbial hangover from alcohol, similar headaches from tablets, excessive smoking, abuse of medicines or drugs may cause headache. Anthony Trollope's bankrupt father deranged his brain and physique through the excessive use of calomel. Today, ergotamines taken in large amounts or constantly without a break of at least two days each week, may cause a prostrating illness with loss of weight, loss of appetite, sleeplessness and depression. Migrainous debility from drugs may prove difficult to treat. Thus, to quote a medical journal: 'The problem may be aggravated by an obstinate refusal to alter an irregular mode of life, coexistent drug addiction, persistent vomiting, refusal to follow instructions or sheer lack of intelligence.' Other headache remedies are sometimes harmful. Many compound preparations taken for headache contain phenacetin. Not only can an excess of phenacetin produce 'rebound' headaches, but phenacetin and/or paracetamol in excess can damage the kidneys. Similarly, aspirin in excess, or taken in small dosages on an empty stomach by certain allergic individuals, can cause bleeding from stomach and bowel.

Headaches with fevers

In general practice, about 10% of headaches for which a doctor is called are associated with fever. They occur mostly in young people and respond to the appropriate treatment. Young females are especially prone to cystitis and pyelitis (bladder and kidney infection) and a dull headache may be a feature of these infections. Headaches may be an early symptom of other infections such as tuberculosis, rickettsial disease in certain countries, leptospirosis, typhoid or food poisoning. These headaches rarely recur and a history of infection is usually obtained. Headaches are often associated with viral illness and may persist for weeks afterwards with a feeling of malaise and depression.

Headaches from anatomical structures

(a) from sinuses
Sinuses are bony, air-filled spaces behind the eye-brows, and behind and to the side of the nose.

Their linings may become congested and, as a result of infection, they may fill with fluid and block, causing a dull pain over the forehead, cheeks or upper teeth. The same areas may be tender to pressure, and pain is often worse on waking and eases towards evening. The eyes may water, the nose may feel blocked, but sensations of sickness or vomiting rarely occur. The pain may be aggravated by the strain of coughing or from wearing a tight collar. The sinuses are particularly sensitive to dust, wind, pollen, fumes or central heating. Congestion of their linings may occur with sexual excitement, menstruation, pregnancy or as a result of over-indulgence, anxiety or frustration. Sinusitis may result from swimming, diving and damp conditions. The presence of moulds in the atmosphere may induce a chronic allergic reaction. Acute sinusitis from sudden changes in barometric pressure may cause discomfort when travelling by aeroplane.

Pain does not always occur with chronic sinusitis, but a state of ill health or anaemia from the chronic infection may trigger other forms of headache. A warning is needed against using nasal decongestants, inhaled or taken as snuff, for if they are taken too frequently they will produce temporary relief at first, but in excess will result in more severe 'rebound' congestion and headache.

Old fashioned remedies, such as the inhalation of hot water vapour steeped in Friar's Balsam (Tinct. Benz. Co.) under a towel may relieve an acute attack following a cold, but more persistent attacks are better referred to a doctor.

(b) from the neck

Many pains arise from the neck with contraction of muscles over the scalp. Such pains may follow injury but are most commonly seen in older people with arthritic changes (spondylosis) in the neck. From around fifty years of age, neck movements become increasingly restricted and muscular head pains arising from the neck are more frequent. They may spread from the back of the head to behind the eyes or to the temples. A host of measures — heat, massage, wearing a surgical collar — may help partially, and tablets to relax muscles may be taken before retiring at night. These tablets may be a most valuable alternative to hypnotics (sleeping tablets).

(c) from the eyes

For those needing glasses a visit to the optician every two years is part of one's personal hygiene. Many pains start round or behind the eye but few, in practice, are related to minor errors in refraction or to squints. Bad lighting conditions —

whether too bright, too dim or the presence of flickering lights — especially at work can induce head pain. In older people, who need to take atropinic drugs or tranquillizers, head pain may indicate the presence of pressure within the eye (glaucoma). The pain comes on gradually, is localized to the eye but may then spread outwards and can be accompanied by nausea and vomiting. Other pains may be associated with disturbances of vision in eye conditions, such as retrobulbar neuritis or uveitis. These conditions require medical attention.

(d) from the ear and bones
Pain may arise from local structures over the face and skull. Parents should be aware that a child with pain around the ear may have an ear infection, tonsillitis or toothache. Local disease of bone can sometimes cause pain in older persons with the occurrence of a dull ache over one eye, perhaps heralding the onset of shingles.

(e) from the teeth and jaw
The pain of migraine is more often projected to the teeth than toothache to the skull, but pains related to muscles and joints of the lower jaw can cause widespread pain in the face and trigger off migraine attacks. The Western European adult

has inherited large facial features from his Nordic ancestors and smaller features from his Mediterranean ancestors. The results, too often, is a misfit between upper and lower teeth, with bad spacing between the teeth and an overhung or underslung, maloccluded jaw. As teeth are sacrificed to over-indulgence in sweets and carbohydrates and replaced by badly fitting dentures, so the lower jaw shrinks and the mechanics of the hinges of the jaw become permanently faulty. Frequent headaches may be the price for such neglect and skilled dental help can be invaluable.

Headaches following injury

A head injury sustained in a game is very often quickly forgotten, whereas a minor knock in other circumstances (particularly at work) may lead to permanent debility. Headaches can follow concussion. There may be tenderness at the site of damage or a steady ache due to spasm and contraction of muscles. Such an ache can arise at the back of the head, spreading forwards, and may result from a severe jolt to the neck. The third type of head pain often comes as attacks of throbbing and aching, often on one side of the head pand associated with giddiness. These episodes of pain may be caused or worsened by noise, excitement, exertion, alcohol or head movement.

A headache soon after an accident, with disabling attacks of dizziness over the next weeks, should gradually lessen in severity. Where this is not so, one of two reasons may well account for its prolongation: either the fear that permanent damage has been done or a resentment related to the circumstances of the accident. The settlement of a long drawn out legal wrangle may well produce a rapid improvement. In my experience, simple treatment and reassurance at an early stage can go far to ease so-called post-traumatic headaches.

In sport, repeated bangs on the head may result in a migraine type of head pain. This is well recorded in the case of footballers who frequently head the ball.

Neurological causes of headache

(a) tumours and abscesses

Concern that frequent headaches may be due to a tumour or an abscess is largely misplaced. In the United Kingdom, ten million people are subject to headaches, yet only 23,000 people develop tumours each year and one never ceases, as a doctor, to be amazed that, whereas people with fevers may firstly complain of a headache, this is rarely so for those found to have tumours. Indeed, where headaches occur, other symptoms overshadow and blunt the individual's awareness of his headpain. Rarely do such pains cause a person to wake. They may build up slowly over several months, are noticed at first on waking but then ease off and perhaps return towards evening. Vomiting, neck stiffness, blunting of interest and alteration of personality will accompany the pain. The active migraine sufferer presents a totally different picture.

(b) bleeds and clots

The bleed of a subarachnoid haemorrhage may come suddenly, perhaps related to exertion. Vomiting usually occurs at the onset of the bleed, commonly followed by loss of temporary alteration of consciousness with an acutely stiff neck, back pain and perhaps some localized numbness or weakness. This is a haemorrhage from blood vessels into the lining membrane and fluid around the brain.

People, particularly the elderly, who receive a severe blow on the head as from an oak beam or a heavy door, may develop a blood clot under the skull and over the surface of the brain (subdural haematoma). Such a person will experience dull head pains, predominantly in the mornings, usually accompanied by a number of mild neurological disturbances such as slight weakness down one side of the body or difficulty with speech. More obviously this pain can be overshadowed by dulling of mental faculties so that the person does not appear to be his normal self over the succeeding week. At any age a good recovery is possible from relatively simple surgical treatment.

(c) arteritis

In people over 60 years of age, the occurrence of a continual dull headache with soreness of the scalp — so that it is painful to wear a hat or comb the hair — weight loss, and if left, loss of vision, may signal cranial arteritis (inflammation of the arteries within the head). There, danger is very real, and urgent referral to a doctor is required.

(d) benign intracranial hypertension

Attacks of severe, recurrent headache, usually accompanied by blurring of vision or double vision, and occurring with weight gain rather than weight loss, may be seen in young women and occasionally in children. It is an uncommon condition which may follow infections, hormonal changes or abnormal reactions to certain drugs. Here the doctor's first concern is to exclude a neurosurgical emergency. Investigations are required, but these headaches, although raising the scare of a tumour, will settle down.

(e) headaches with epilepsy

As a person starts to recover from a convulsion, he may pass through a stage of disorientation and is then left with drowsiness and headache. The headache of epilepsy is almost invariably following repeated sensations or movements, usually with loss or alteration of consciousness. Compared with focal migraine in which the march of sensations develop over several minutes, the abnormal sensations or movements of epilepsy develop and spread within a few seconds.

(f) neuralgias

Periodic migrainous neuralgia, also known as cluster or clock headaches, will be discussed as a variant of migraine. Trigemminal neuralgia (*tic douloureux*) is a pain confined to the face and mouth, and inevitably requires medical attention to separate it from other pains in the face. It tends not to respond to simple analgesic tablets and special treatment is required. Your dentist will be able to distinguish it from various pains around the teeth and his help can be invaluable.

VARIETIES OF MIGRAINE

Common migraine

This is the term used when a headache, recurring at intervals, usually affects half the head and is accompanied by eye disturbances or sickness. One in 10 people are prone to common migraine, less than 1 in 50 liable to classical migraine and the more complicated forms of migraine, though well recognized, are very rare.

Classical migraine

This is the term used when the symptoms of unilateral headache are preceded by warning signs such as disturbed vision, taking such forms as zigzags, brightly coloured spots or islands of visual loss. These symptoms occur with constriction of blood vessels and often last for 10–30 minutes before the onset of the headache. They are referred to as focal symptoms and point anatomically to the blood vessels primarily involved. The sheer complexity of the possible phenomena is of great interest to neurologists but rarely has any permanent significance.

Focal migraine

This term is often used when focal symptoms overshadow the actual headache attacks. The visual symptoms may be quite dramatic with brightly scintillating shimmering or coloured blobs causing patches of visual loss. Vision may be lost to one side, at the sides, or altitudinally. The disturbances may appear hallucinatory with objects appearing larger, smaller or, as a mosaic, like broken coloured pebbles. Colours may be heightened or objects appear strange or unduly familiar. Double vision or drooping of the eyelid can occur. With retinal migraine loss of vision in one eye may be followed by a headache localized to the affected eye. With other types of focal attacks, speech may be affected with the words slurred or jumbled. One half of the body or part of the face may go numb or weak (hemianaesthetic, hemiparetic or facial migraine, respectively) and characteristically the headache occurs on the same side as the focal symptoms. Such symptoms may persist for up to 30 minutes and then clear. Amigranous migraine is the term used when focal symptoms develop without any subsequent headache.

Complicated migraine

More persistent symptoms may occur with hemiplegic, facioplegic or ophthalmoplegic migraine. These forms are often familiar and follow a course typical for that family. Hemiplegic migraine may produce a weakness which clears within hours or persists for nearly two weeks. At least two different forms of this condition are known. Facial weakness, with drooping of part of the face, occurs in facioplegic migraine; and with ophthalmoplegic migraine — seen in less than 1 in 500 migraine sufferers — double vision or inequality of the pupils from weakness or paralysis of the eye muscles may persist for weeks after the headache has cleared. Very rarely, indeed, do such symptoms become permanent, but doctors recognize the need for reassurance and are prepared to use various non-invasive tests by way of reassurance.

Basilar migraine

Named after the basilar artery supplying the back part of the brain, this is most frequently seen in adolescent girls and young adults and has a strong menstrual association. Initially, there may be dimming or loss of vision, or flashes and blobs of black or white, so intense as to blot out vision. Giddiness, a metallic taste, unsteadiness, noises in the head, slurred speech and tingling of the hands, feet or around the mouth, may be followed by a severe headache. At the height of the attack, consciousness may be lost. The loss of consciousness is no way epileptic but due to the migraine.

Migrainous equivalents

These are a variety of symptoms which may replace the more usual migraine attack. In childhood cyclic vomiting is well known to paediatricians and in adults may be replaced by bilious attacks of abdominal migraine. Periodic diarrhoea, fever, palpitations or chest pains may just occasionally have a migrainous basis, but it is a diagnosis made by the doctor only after he is convinced that alternative explanations have been excluded.

Periodic migrainous neuralgia

Also known as cluster headaches, clock headaches and by a host of other names, this affects males more often than females, and has a very characteristic form. Paroxysms of pain of agonizing severity occur around or behind the eye and last two hours or less. They may, during the course of six weeks, occur with clockwork precision once or twice every 24 hours, and after the bout has ended complete relief follows for rarely less than six months and perhaps for several years. Alcohol is a very definite precipitant of an attack during the course of a bout of neuralgia, but in general the causation of attacks is poorly understood. Standard migraine therapy is inadequate in periodic migrainous neuralgia and it is wisest to consult one's doctor.

The severity of the attack may be such that your doctor may give you a pain-killing injection, perhaps using a morphine derivative, but the most effective treatment for severe attacks is the injection intramuscularly of Femergin (0.5mg) or dihydroergotamine (2mg) an hour or so before the expected time of the attack. Patients are often taught to give their own injections. For more chronic migrainous neuralgia, methysergide (Deseril, 1mg three times daily), taken by mouth, may prove successful, but this drug should never be taken for more than 4–6 weeks at a time.

Icepick headaches

Named after the stiletto-like instrument used to pick out lumps of ice when preparing cocktails, this refers to periodic sharp, lancinating head pains, usually of brief duration. There is a possible association with migraine but the pains are essentially innocent, harmless and too short-lived to require specific treatment.

THE SO-CALLED 'ORDINARY' HEADACHE

It will already be apparent that a brief, mild or nondescript headache is most probably a minor form of tension headache, produced by contraction of the scalp, temporal and neck muscles. Such headaches may also be felt before changes in the weather — a barometer before thunder or portending the onset of damp or humid conditions. Some complain of headache due to overwork. It is the monotony of the routine or the dreary nature of the task rather than the time and effort expended which more usually is responsible for such headaches. Eye-strain from close work, as when reading, may in part be caused by refractory errors and astigmatism; but the importance of these factors is often overplayed and minor errors of astigmatism seem to be of far greater concern to the inhabitants of the United Kingdom than to those of any other nation. Equally important in the eye-strain headache is the quality of the lighting and the anxiety pressures involved in the task.

Anxiety headaches may appear as a 'conditioned reflex response' when something unexpected happens. Paul Gallico's cat would respond to any new situation by stopping, washing, and would then survey the scene. How sensible! Too many people respond to the unexpected with a brief headache and if, on a particular occasion, the headache is not forthcoming, almost wish one on themselves. Other anxiety headaches arise as a response to inbred fears or phobias, such as the fear of confined spaces (claustrophia).

A very real headache may arise in the stuffy atmosphere of a car if the amount of carbon monoxide, leaking from the engine, is allowed to build up inside. A headache may arise when in an over-heated room, where the central heating has dried the atmosphere. Sinusitis experienced on moving to a damp river valley or wet coastal plain can produce a headache which may be further intensified by repeated sneezing. The sinusitis can be allergic or seasonal with the presence of moulds and other spores in the air. The relation of headache, anaemia and infection has already been discussed. Similar headaches can arise from constipation. The treatment is not from yet more constipating tablets but from attention to a proper proportion of roughage, such as bran, in the diet. Any tablets, especially barbiturates, but also including tranquillizers, anti-tension drugs such as valium, and even antibiotics, can cause headaches as an unavoidable side effect. In general, combinations of tablets are more prone to cause headaches than single tablets. Even tablets taken specifically for headache relief may cause a rebound headache when overused or abused.

I was especially requested to comment on the 'everyday' headache. Implicit in the term is the suggestion that a headache can be expected 'everyday'. As readers will have realized already, such a term is never a diagnosis. No headache is inevitable. By a careful analysis of the possible causes — basically something which only the sufferer can do, though often with the help and guidance of others — a more accurate diagnosis leading to a course of action is possible. To those who still believe in the 'everyday' headache, I would pose four questions:

(a) Is the answer to your problem psychological? Have you allowed yourself to become over-anxious, tense, or a moaner, and is this attitude in any way good for you or helpful? Perhaps a discussion with a friend or the development of a new interest would be helpful.

(b) Are you taking too many tablets or too many different types of tablets?

(c) Have you allowed your bowel and eating habits to become irregular? It is probable that a spoonful of bran with the breakfast cereal cures far more headaches than a weekly bottle of aspirin.

(d) Are you using your headache as a means of escape from a difficult situation? Remember that a pain in the head is never appreciated by others. Do not wear yourself out attempting to make others sympathize and appreciate the presence of your head pain.

MIGRAINE IN CHILDREN

People often fail to appreciate that migraine can start early in life. Children may have migraine attacks, rendering them cross and irritable, every bit as bad or prolonged as in adult life. There are three specific types of attack observed mainly in childhood.

Before the age of 10, a child may be subject to frequent attacks of 'indigestion' and 'biliousness', during which he becomes fretful and irritable with crying and vomiting. After the vomiting, he is then more comfortable, may go off to sleep and waken quite well. This is cyclic vomiting.

Secondly, a child may experience severe but disconcertingly brief headaches lasting

10–30 minutes, and yet before and after the event he may play, jump and shout with impunity.

Thirdly, there is a rare form seen mainly in childhood consisting of hallucinations in which the size or shape of the body is distorted — the Alice in Wonderland, or Alice and the Mushroom disorder. I can quote the experience of an adult, a lady of 20 who, whilst sitting having tea, stretched out her right hand and thought it seemed to have grown. She could not see to her right or her children on the settee. Then the arm, from elbow to finger tips, appeared numb and her speech went garbled. The right side of her mouth went dead, though later the symptoms improved, the thumb being the last to recover. The whole episode lasted 20–30 minutes. Finally, she had a headache over the right temple which lasted until the next day. Would your child, if he or she attempted to relate such an experience, be told to shut up?

What to do with migraine in childhood

In the school room or at home, the best treatment is to let a child lie down in a darkened room until the attack passes off. Loss from school or classes should be minimized. Although a junior aspirin may be helpful for the longer attack, there is little point in attempting to treat the shorter episode. Some explanation of the forms of treatment used by doctors to prevent attacks in childhood may be of help. Anti-sickness tablets may be given once or twice a day, especially when sickness or nausea comes with the headache, but one of the more popular preparations — Maxalon — is avoided in childhood as it can lead to unexpected reactions. Mild anticonvulsants, such as phenobarbitone, may be used and indeed the doctor may order an electro-encephalogram (brain wave test), not to exclude epilepsy, but to check whether such tablets may be useful. Allergic factors can be associated with childhood migraine, especially in a child with asthma and travel sickness, but dietary factors — apart from ice-cream, which induces a particular headache related to its coldness — rarely give rise to migraine in children.

Preparing for exams

Headaches when swotting for an exam, and the fear of headache during an exam, affect children and adults alike. Over-sedation with drugs should always be avoided, and untried drugs, which may have the wrong effect on an individual, never used. Students, in particular, should plan a careful schedule. Continued swotting for long hours produces a diminishing return. Over-indulgence in coffee, tea or cigarettes should be avoided and frequent intervals taken for a rest, a walk, a proper meal and for sleep. A clear programme of work, rather then chasing a wild goal, is important. In reading each chapter, pick out the three or four salient points, decide why these points are important, how they interrelate and how other aspects of the chapter embellish these key points. If, after avoiding the likely triggers of a migraine attack, you are still worried about the possibility of migraine, see your doctor. Student Health Centres have become especially skilled at advising people in this situation.

MIGRAINE IN WOMEN

Menstrual migraine

Attacks predominantly at period times occur in 14% of women subject to migraine and may be associated with weight gain and breast discomfort. There is no specific hormonal change to account for menstrual migraine but hormonal therapy is occasionally justified. Orthodox treatments for migraine are just as effective in menstrual migraine. It is advisable to avoid excessive salt and fluid intake in the days before the period starts, i.e. avoid adding salt to cooked food, limit the salt when cooking vegetables and limit the number of beverages taken. The use of diuretic tablets (to increase the output of urine) to prevent migraine has proved disappointing in the main. Most forms of menstrual migraine improve during pregnancy or at the menopause.

Migraine at the menopause

Most forms of headache may worsen temporarily at the menopause. Afterwards migraine tends to improve. Tension factors and depression must always be considered.

Migraine in pregnancy

Eighty per cent of women with migraine have fewer attacks during pregnancy. The improvement is maintained throughout the pregnancy, but attacks may return after childbirth. Only occasionally does migraine actually worsen during pregnancy. Pregnant women are aware of the dangers of medication that might affect the unborn child. Ergot preparations and Deseril (methysergide) should be avoided absolutely. Salt and fluid should be watched carefully and little salt added to food. Headaches are less likely if a positive state of physical and mental well-being is maintained throughout pregnancy, and simple measures to avoid morning sickness and vomiting may help. On waking a water biscuit or piece of dry toast can be taken before getting up slowly. Avoid the tendency to linger in bed all day and keep a regular, bright and busy routine. Fresh interests are important, particularly for a person who has been busy until the start of the pregnancy. Fatty food, too much butter or milk, should be avoided at breakfast, and hot or cold drinks may best be taken half an hour before meals rather than with the meal.

Migraine and contraception

Migraine as such does not contra-indicate the use of the contraceptive pill. Indeed, many migraine sufferers have fewer attacks whilst on the pill and their anxieties are relieved. The pill is best avoided in persons with thrombotic tendencies, active liver disease, cancer, undiagnosed vaginal bleeding or raised blood pressure. With the replacement of the high-dose oestrogen pill by that with a lower oestrogen content, or by the progesterone-alone pill, the risk of thromboses has been greatly reduced. Some women experience other, less severe side effects such as tension, tiredness, weight gain and changes in libido which may catch up on them surreptitiously and worsen their migraine; but these symptoms can often be alleviated by changing the brand of pill. There are, however, certain circumstances when it is advisable to stop oral contraceptives and not to restart later:

(1) if the first attack of migraine occurs on starting the pill
(2) if there is a dramatic increase in the number of attacks
(3) if the character of the attacks changes, becoming more focal, e.g. involving specific parts of the face or limbs
(4) if any form of thrombosis develops.

The success of other forms of contraception may depend on their aesthetic appeal and freedom from anxiety. Occasionally the coil (intrauterine contraceptive device) may increase menstrual loss and worsen headache by causing anaemia. For a woman who has fulfilled her matrimonial ambitions after successful childbirth, sterilization is acceptable, but if performed for the wrong reasons may leave a legacy of psychological problems precipitating any headache tendency. (The same advice holds true with respect to vasectomy in men.)

MIGRAINE AND SEX

Two aspects of sex and migraine may cause concern. Firstly, with the tendency for migraine to alter the distribution of fluid within the body there may be surges of sensations involving the sex parts, often with an increase in sex drive. Increased sexual activity in relation to migraine is essentially harmless, and indeed the exertion involved may bring relief for some individuals. Secondly, quite separately from any migraine tendency, some people may experience head pain with intercourse. The pain is due to raised pressure within the head and in this respect is similar to cough headache. People are sometimes concerned that they may have had a small bleed within the head, but this is unlikely unless the head pain is accompanied by vomiting, neck stiffness and other features. Problems caused by infertility in one or both partners, or the fear of venereal disease which is on the increase throughout the world, are prime examples of tension factors which often remain undisclosed.

MIGRAINE IN OLDER PEOPLE

The tendency to migraine declines with age. It is rare for migraine to develop for the first time after the age of 45, and it is advisable to seek other explanations (most of which have already been discussed in the earlier pages) before accepting migraine as the sole cause of worsening headaches after 55 years of age.

LOSS OF CONSCIOUSNESS WITH MIGRAINE

Basilar migraine is recognized as a cause of temporary loss of consciousness and predominantly affects healthy young women. Other forms of migraine are occasionally associated with fainting, but epilepsy does not occur with any greater frequency in the migraineur.

CONFUSION AND MIGRAINE

A person with partial loss of vision and reduced oxygen to part of the brain may feel confused. The individual usually feels more confused than his actions suggest and is never likely to commit an impulsive act. There are other causes of temporary lack of awareness, forgetfulness or confusion and it would be wise to consult one's doctor. In the older textbooks, the term 'status hemicranicus' was used to describe a rapid sequence of migraine attacks from which the sufferer receives no respite. As more is known about migraine, and particularly about alternative diagnoses and the dangers of over-medication, this is no longer an acceptable diagnosis without detailed medical examination.

DRIVING AND MIGRAINE

Migraine sufferers are rarely prevented on medical grounds from driving altogether, but there are many circumstances when a migraineur should be aware that he cannot drive with complete safety and should refrain from driving until his attacks are under control. Guidance is given in the pamphlet *Medical Aspects of Fitness to Drive* prepared by the Medical Commission on Accident Prevention.

Driving may be rendered hazardous by:
  (1) loss or alteration of consciousness
  (2) confusional states — the result of vascular changes, pain or medication
  (3) giddiness or vertigo
  (4) double vision
  (5) total or partial loss of vision — people are not always aware of binocular loss of vision or loss of vision to one side or in one quadrant.

If any of these disabling features occur during your attacks, or if an attack is more severe than usual, you should stop driving immediately the warning signs appear. In the United States, a lorry driver on a five-lane highway developed total blindness during a migraine attack and was guided to safety by a passing car using citizens band (C.B.) radio. Often an attack may develop in a busy thoroughfare or on a motorway.

If the onset of the attack is signalled by double vision, it may be possible, covering one eye, to drive to a safe stopping place. On the motorway, an emergency stop on the hard shoulder is permitted in the case of sudden illness. However, it is necessary to emphasize that a lot of motorway accidents occur due to vehicles stopping on the hard shoulder and it is a risky place to be, particularly if you are not feeling well. When moving off from the hard shoulder it is quite difficult to judge the speed of vehicles travelling in the slow lane. Furthermore, the police will not take a lenient view of someone who attempts to sleep off a migraine attack on the hard shoulder. In a town it may be even more difficult to make an emergency stop. Do not do so on the approach to a pedestrian crossing. Although one may be liable to prosecution, if it is necessary to park on a double yellow line, or elsewhere contrary to the highway code, most authorities will listen to an explanation of ill-health due to migraine, and a medical report in mitigation may well carry the day.

A person with frequent attacks is strongly advised not to drive; thus women with premenstrual migraine should not drive at the relevant times. Fortunately, hormonal therapy has reduced the number of women whose attacks are regularly and distressingly disabling. Anyone taking drugs, especially for the first time, should be particularly careful and, if possible, should avoid driving. Unfortunately, research on the effect of drugs on driving has not kept pace with modern prescribing. Antihistamines and antidepressives are recognized as potentially hazardous, particularly in combination with other drugs, and there may be unexpected side effects, for example, methyldopa given to lower blood pressure may also induce drowsiness. Alcohol should never be taken with other drugs and anyone driving in such circumstances can expect to be punished.

Tinted lenses and tinted windscreens may present quite a problem whilst driving, particularly to those without perfect sight. A tinted lens on average can restrict the acuity of vision by 7%. The same applies to a tinted windscreen so that the cumulative effect may be a 14% reduction in vision which may prove dangerous whilst driving at night and trying to peer into the shadows of the glare from oncoming headlights. Polaroid glasses will reduce glare but photochromic glasses will not.

Lastly, anyone driving should attempt to avoid any of the known precipitating causes of migraine, for example:

(1) fatigue — by not driving long periods without rest
(2) bright sunlight — by using Polaroid glasses
(3) a low blood sugar (hypoglycaemia) — by having regular frequent meals.

Travel and migraine

Many adult migraineurs find that if they drive they are less liable to attacks of migraine or travel sickness and can adjust the heating and ventilation to their own liking. Children and other passengers are less fortunate. For a long journey, cyclizine taken half an hour beforehand may be helpful. Light but frequent meals should be taken and there should be breaks in the journey to stretch their legs, sight-see and avoid monotony and fatugue.

Care should be taken not to overload the inside of the car. The passenger space and rear window should be as uncluttered as possible to allow adequate ventilation, avoid dust, and prevent the accumulation of carbon monoxide — which is itself a potent cause of headache. The migraine or travel-sick child should never sit at the back of a bus but as close to the driver as possible.

THE IMPORTANCE OF TRIGGER FACTORS WHICH PRODUCE ATTACKS

Why do attacks of migraine happen at certain times? We may examine the possible factors which may trigger off a migraine attack. If such precipitants can be removed or avoided, there is a chance of reducing the number of attacks. It may be worth keeping a migraine diary. A record can be built up of the days and times of the onset of attacks. The same precipitant will probably not explain every attack. There may be a diversity of causes and in good time the individual might show a resistance to a trigger factor which undoubtedly would cause an attack on a more vulnerable occasion. Recognition and awareness of trigger factors might confer a substantial benefit on the well-being of the sufferer.

The more common types of precipitants can be summarized under the following headings:

Psychological and emotional factors

These include emotion, anxiety, depression, shock and excitement. If these are recognized, the migraineur can be forearmed. One cannot always avoid anxiety or over-excitement, but faced with states of emotional excitement one can take greater care to avoid other factors which might also provoke migraine, thus 'removing the fuse from the shell'. One may consciously alter one's attitude to emotional problems and situations, making light of them or steeling oneself to the possible consequences. On a doctor's advice, the use of a simple tranquillizer might lessen the impact of the emotional affront. Do not allow one's subconscious to manipulate the situation. For example, do not attempt to seek the gratification of martyrdom by claiming the privileges of an invalid. Be cautious, too, lest the headache is an expression of a basic feeling of insecurity when striving to attempt too much or attempting more than you really feel psychologically up to. I have added these last two sentences to prevent the type of introspection which might set a vicious cycle of headache and anxiety state.

Alterations in health

Recurrent health problems — anaemia from heavy periods, bouts of cystitis, sinusitis and 'flu, or toothache — tend to become a bore and a nuisance. The temptation is to attempt to shrug such troubles off and, rather than be accused of hypochondriasis, to disregard health problems which may also trigger off migraine attacks. If there is any connection between such problems and migraine, there is even more reason to treat them seriously and to seek medical advice and effective treatment.

Menstrual factors

Premenstrual tension or the onset of the meno-pause are potent triggers of attacks. They have already been discussed in the appropriate sections of the book.

Fatigue

Mental fatigue may take several forms: working against a deadline, overstimulation of the senses of hearing, sight or smell, prolonged focusing on work, TV or the cinema screen, failure to relax mentally before travelling, or the struggle to keep going in the face of psychological problems.

Physical fatigue can come from over-exertion or from more specific forms of exertion, such as stooping for long periods or lifting heavy weights. Fatigue of any type brings to light all the subconscious tension factors. If physical fatigue is recognized as a factor, the remedies are usually fairly easy to apply. Examine whether the tasks can be done with better posture, e.g. kneeling rather than stooping or bending the knees and not the back to move furniture, etc. Mental fatigue is not always recognized but check whether:

(a) your friends comment that you always look serious and worried

(b) you find yourself clenching your jaws, grinding your teeth or making a tight fist with your hands, or

(c) have you sought dental aid because your teeth are tender or chipped?

If forms of fatigue are recognized as definite triggers, one may plan a routine which avoids boredom, repetition or exhaustion and can protect oneself by developing means of relaxation.

Changes in routine

Migraineurs can be divided into those who have the majority of their attacks when under pressure, as when trying to complete a task against a deadline, and those who suffer from 'let down' headaches, particularly when they try to relax at weekends. The weekend headache may be triggered by a number of factors. Many migraine sufferers find that a set routine is helpful in keeping themselves occupied and their energies directed. Secondly, they may have difficulty adjusting to a change in routine, e.g. from the demands of the office to the demands of the family. Similarly, holidays or a change in shift work may precipitate headaches. And thirdly, the weekend may involve irregular meal times, dietary indiscretions, the hangover effect of sleeping tablets, especially taken on top of alcohol, late rising after prolonged sleep, concurrent hypoglycaemia (low blood sugar due to a delayed breakfast), and sleeping in an overheated bedroom. These factors may prove particularly irksome to those migraineurs with obsessional traits and it may even be necessary to provide some sort of planned routine for the weekend.

Environmental factors

The question is often asked whether changes in weather can cause migraine. Undoubtedly extremes of climate with little chance for acclimatization, high winds, dust storms, smoke, dazzling sunlight and humid conditions may all produce headaches. Conditions at work may have a similar effect. Poor lighting, too strong lighting, fluorescent or flickering lights, noise levels, high pitched sounds, dusts, chemicals and even domestic gas are recognized as potential triggers. People working with chemicals have been known to change their clothing and wash their hair each day on returning home to prevent other members of the family developing headaches.

Allergies

Children with asthma or other alergic manifestations which respond to specific therapy may develop migraine when their primary allergy is brought under control. Household pets may be a source of allergy. Many children and adults find that their headaches are controlled by antihistamines and desensitization can be beneficial.

Dietary factors

Certain specific foods, notably chocolate, cheese, citrus fruits (oranges, lemons, grapefruits) and alcohol can provoke attacks in about one-third of migraineurs. An equally potent cause of migraine may be missing meals, irregular meals or fasting.

An adequate breakfast or a small cooked meal at mid-day may prevent the onset of attacks. Over-indulgence in spiced foods, alcohol, tea, coffee, tobacco and even compulsive water drinking may, on occasion, provoke attacks.

DIET AND HEADACHE

Physicians are forever anxious to avoid the prescription of unnecessary diets. They are taught that over-hasty and unreasonable prohibition of a patient's pleasures does no good. The pliable are made wretched, but most are merely alienated. Shakespeare expressed the same notion in the words of Falstaff:

If sack and sugar be a fault. God help the wicked!
If to be old and merry be a sin, then many an old host that I know is damn'd;
If to be fat be to be hated, then Pharaoh's lean kine are to be loved.

Thus, although there are dangers in over-indulgence and obesity, a balance must be struck, and it is moderation not parsimony for which one must aim. Likewise, it is necessary to retain a sense of proportion in discussing diet and headache. Certain chemicals added to food as preservatives can often precipitate headache.

They can be listed, and they can be avoided without seriously affecting one's normal food intake. However, the question of food allergy and migraine has been overplayed. Only a third of adults prone to migraine, and very few children, have a definite food allergy which during vulnerable times can cause headache. In practice it is not easy to establish that a particular food causes a headache in a susceptible individual. There are enthusiasts for food allergies who claim that it is possible to tell whether an allergy exists from alterations in mood, blood pressure, tension and fatiguability after sampling a small quantity of a possible allergen (i.e. something which could cause an allergy), but this approach has been rightly condemned as unscientific and in reality only tests the extent to which the particular individual is of an anxious disposition.

A second myth which needs to be exploded is that salads, vegetables and fruit can cause headache because they contain acid. This myth is a hangover from a belief that roughage in the diet has no useful function and that anything with coarse fibre is 'hardly the food for a lady'. The reverse has been shown to be the case. Roughage can prevent some bleeding conditions related to menstruation and child birth. More so, the great advance over the past decade in medicine applied to the digestive system has been the recognition of the importance of dietary fibre (roughage) as an essential ingredient in a proper diet. The story began with the observation that adequate roughage in the diet of sailors avoided the need to deal out pills for constipation. Since then the occurence of various diseases — piles, gall-bladder disorders, diverticulitis, appendicitis and cystitis — have been related throughout the world to the average intake of dietary fibres by the inhabitants of various countries and differences between the different racial groups and what they eat. Over-indulgence in refined carbohydrates in the Western World and among the better off in India and the Far East has also been accompanied by an increase in raised blood pressure, coronary heart disease and arteriosclerosis.

These facts have a practical bearing on the causation of headaches. Unrefined carbohydrates, for example in vegetable foods and unsophisticated flour, are slowly absorbed; and the roughage they contain is able to bind potential poisons and hold them within the intestine. The more bulky bowel contents improve the muscular tone of the bowel and help establish regular bowel habits. Constipation, which is a cause of headache, is lessened. The constipating effect of medicines taken for headache is also reduced.

Sources of infection, such as diverticulitis, which can be responsible for recurrent bowel, bladder and kidney infections, are removed and the person is less likely to become mildly anaemic.

All that needs to be advocated to establish a healthy diet is:

(a) a sensible reduction in the amount of refined foods taken each day, e.g. granulated sugar, cakes and prepared foods
(b) a switch from white to brown breads
(c) the addition of a small amount of bran along with one's breakfast cereal
(d) a regular intake of fruit, root vegetables and salads.

I am prepared to accept that to take fruit occasionally, if one is unused to such foods, may cause indigestion, but taken along with the above diet, the chances of being upset by the 'acidity' of food is something which the headache sufferer need fear no longer.

FOOD AND MIGRAINE

There have been two most thorough scientific studies by Dr E. Hanington and Dr K. Dalton into dietary factors which people recognize as likely to precipitate migrainous attacks. In Dr

Hanington's study she found that of 500 migraineurs the following proportions avoided:

Chocolate	74%
Cheese and dairy products	47%
Fruit, particularly citrus fruit	30%
Alcohol	25%
Fried fatty foods	18%
Vegetables	18%
Tea and coffee	15%
Meat, particularly pork	14%
Sea food, e.g. shell fish	10%

With respect to alcohol, many find that white
wine agrees better than red, and spirits more so
than wines or aperitifs. The hot, noisy and smoky
atmosphere of a cocktail party and the delayed
time of eating may be factors inducing an attack.

Certain chemical substances liable to cause
headaches have been identified in particular foods.

Chemical	*Food*
Tyramine	in pickled herrings, yeast extracts such as marmite, and cheeses, especially more mature cheeses such as Brie, Camembert and Stilton

Betaphenylethylamine — in chocolate
Histamine — in cheeses and drinks
Octopamine — in citrus fruits
5 hydroxytryptamine — in tomatoes, pineapples, bananas
Monosodium glutamate (symptoms include headache, burning feeling in the face, sensation of pressure on the chest). — used as flavour enhancer especially in Chinese restaurants, Japanese sukiyaki, Kosher chicken soup, Matzo ball soup, Green pea soup
Sodium nitrite
'Hot dog headache' — in frankfurters, bacon, cured meats, e.g. salami, hot dogs.

How to eliminate dietary factors

If you are concerned that your headache may have a dietary basis:

(1) keep a diary of foods and where eaten
(2) stop the foods most liable to cause headache, e.g. chocolate, cheeses, spiced or prepared foods and heavy wines for at least six weeks
(3) over the next six weeks avoid citrus fruits, coffee and fried foods

(4) if really necessary, try an elimination schedule, limiting yourself for 2 days at a time to:
one beverage, e.g. coffee, tea, water or juices;
and try taking coffee and tea without milk;
one type of meat, e.g. chicken, lamb, turkey,
ham, pork; one vegetable in addition to pota-
toes.

Even during this trial period, carbohydrates,
breads, non-citrus fruit and fish may be taken in
normal quantities. Dairy products should be
watched and care taken to ensure that meals,
however unappetizing, are taken regularly.

Self-help in migraine

The purpose of this booklet on migraine and
headaches has been to provide a practical guide
and to remove the mystery surrounding a condition that affects 8–10% of people. Most migraine
sufferers are aware that 2 out of every 3 migraineurs can be helped by self-help and self-
analysis, as shown by Dr H.G. Wolff in his
classical work, *Headache and Other Head Pain*,
first published in 1948: 'The patient must appreciate that anything out of a bottle can offer no more
than transient help . . . The long term aim should
be to help the individual understand the basis of

his tensions, the factors in his life that aggravate it and to aid him in resolving his conflicts.'

To agree with this view is not to claim that 90% of head pains are psychological. It is to recognize that self-help has an important role. However, as a doctor, one is also aware that headaches cannot be dismissed as inevitably 'of the mind', and specific medical treatment has an important and vital supporting role. Modern medicine is built on the realization that the sufferer has the right to know, and that his knowledge of his personal complaint should be as full as humanly possible:
— so that he can make fine adjustments to his treatment and know the possible consequences of his actions
— so that he may thus achieve a state of positive health, despite his complaint, know how to avoid circumstances which may bring on the trouble, how to take evasive action at the onset of an attack and mitigate the later consequences
— thus, his doctor becomes a friend and adviser rather than a witch doctor, conjuror or disciplinarian.

GUIDE TO TREATMENT

(1) Self-analysis — awareness of causes of migraine; migraine tendencies and traits.

(2) Treatment without drugs — maintaining good general health; avoiding triggers; relaxation therapy — biofeedback, hypnosis, yoga, meditation, Zen; acupuncture.
(3) Non-medical forms of treatment — herbal; combatting the acute attack.
(4) Value of drugs — at the time of an attack; drugs obtained across the counter; drugs on prescription; drugs taken regularly to prevent attacks developing.

Self analysis

It is hoped that this book has already provided the opportunity to study the various types of headache, how they can interrelate and how head pains can be brought on. The questions covered would otherwise require several prolonged interviews with a doctor or therapist. It may still be helpful to discuss those aspects of the problem which appear to affect you, personally, whether with your doctor or with a confidant.

Migraine can afflict anyone — brilliant individuals and those of low intelligence, the obsessional and the sloppy, the energetic and the lethargic. A proportion of those with migraine do possess the neat, obsessional, migrainous personality that has tended to be romanticized in the past. There is much to commend in the migrainous personality, certainly as far as society is concerned, but unfortunately this type of personality can pose many problems and it may be helpful in self-analysis to examine the underside of the coin.

One aspect of the personality is a striving for perfection, a fight to attain the highest standards and, even when such standards are achieved, the individual is rarely satisfied with the result. Failure often engenders guilt. There is an intolerance not only of one's own imperfections, permitting no excuse, but also an intolerance of others, making little allowance for physical or mental inadequacies and not surprisingly leading to conflicts. Obsessional time-keeping of appointments or schedules with a work ethic which despises slowness and idleness may lead to unnecessary irritation. Tension may show in the voice. Feelings of guilt, compulsion or resentment may arise from failure to achieve standards indoctrinated or inculcated by a hypercritical parent, often possessing the same obsessional traits. Self-reproach from irritation or failure to meet a standard may result in exacerbations of migraine.

Treatment without drugs

The importance of general health and avoiding migraine triggers has already been stressed. Let us concentrate now upon the fact that relaxation works and discuss how it can be achieved. Yoga, Zen and Transcendental Meditation can be regarded as directed relaxation, i.e. relaxation with a further goal. Hypnosis and biofeedback depend upon the application of medical techniques to improve relaxation. There are various forms of biofeedback: patients can be trained to increase skin temperatures in the hand in relation to the forehead, and use this to abort headaches; they can observe the state of tension within their frontal and temporal muscles and learn how to relax these muscles; or they can observe how the brain wave patterns (electroencephalographic patterns) can alter from a pattern of arousal, with suppressed alpha activity and increased beta (fast) activity, to one of relaxation with a well developed alpha rhythm. These are feedback devices to show the person's state of relaxation and to teach him how further relaxation can be obtained. The success of such devices has been examined scientifically and it has been shown from a five-year follow-up study that biofeedback is most successful with females under 30 years of age, not habituated to medication, without depressive symptoms and diagnosed as suffering from vascular headaches, i.e. biofeedback is as successful with migraine headaches as with muscular contraction headaches.

Simple forms of relaxation, performed alone or as group therapy, may achieve similar results. Firstly, twenty minutes should be set aside regularly, twice a day, for uninterrupted relaxation. A ritual of relaxation should be followed. Lie down on a couch and note the state of tension of your muscles. Notice your right foot, tense the muscles, then let them relax and go as floppy as possible. Repeat the manoeuvre with your left foot, calf muscles, thighs, abdominal muscles, right hand — make a fist, then relax it — left hand — likewise — elbows and shoulders. Is your jaw clenched? Relax it. Relax your face and your throat. Press your head against the cushion, then relax the neck muscles. Turn your attention to your breathing. Let it become quiet, rhythmical and slow. Ease it still further. Try and appreciate the feeling of relaxation.

Acupuncture achieves much the same result. The treatment needs to be done regularly for at least six weeks. The limiting factor is that the services of those expert in acupuncture — which has many other applications to painful conditions

— is already overstretched and the use of acu-puncture in migraine is very demanding on the time of the therapist.

Non medical forms of treatment

(a) Herbal
The weed or herb, Feverfew, has been publicized for the treatment of migraine, and over the cen-turies many herbal remedies have been developed but there has been no scientific appraisal of their worth.

(b) Combatting the acute attack
The ideal method of combatting an attack is to take analgesic tablets, lie down in a darkened room and sleep it off. This treatment is not always possible. Woken by a headache in the middle of the night, many find it helpful to douche their head in cold water or even to take a cold bath or shower. Some people deliberately undertake vigorous exercise, and Wolff mentions that stand-ing on the head improves vasoconstrictive re-flexes in scalp arteries and has a rational basis for the gymnastically adroit! Others find solace in drinking cups of warm tea. It rarely helps to attempt to make oneself vomit in order to abort the attack; and there is no value in attempting to

fight off the attack for hours before taking tablets. If tablets are taken in migraine they should be taken as early as possible at the beginning of an attack, or else the chances are that they will not be absorbed and will prove ineffective.

The technique of auto-acupuncture has been developed to help ward off a migraine attack where it is not possible to take tablets. The thumb-nail is dug into the skin over various pressure points: on the side of the hand half way between the base of the index finger and the wrist; at the top of the nose between the eyes; below the eyes on each cheek; above the eyes over the eyebrows; just above the outer angles of the eyes; and on either side of the back of the neck. The technique is surprisingly simple to apply. It is also possible at the height of an attack to relieve pain by injecting pressure points about the head with a local anaesthetic agent. The injection will be painful at first until the anaesthetic takes effect.

The value of drugs

At the beginning of an attack
— medicines obtained across the counter
— medicines on prescription
Taken regularly to prevent attacks developing (prophylactic drugs).

The person who has occasional attacks has every right to indulge himself by taking the appropriate drugs and then going to lie down and sleep off the attack. The attack may serve as a warning to ease up temporarily. When attacks occur in inappropriate circumstances and it is not possible to relax or take things easy for a while, medicines are the only effective form of treatment. With a child or young adult, it is important to realize that the person really does have a headache, even if there is an obvious psychological cause, and the headache should be treated seriously as with any other medical condition. It is only when headaches start to occur too frequently, are too persistent and take too much of a toll of one's life and that of one's family or friends, that a more searching analysis becomes of paramount importance.

The basic treatment of a migraine attack is to take one or two tablets of a simple analgesic drug, such as aspirin or paracetamol, as soon as the attack begins. The tablets can then be repeated every two hours until the attack subsides. More sophisticated combined tablets may contain a mixture of analgesics or an analgesic combined with a stimulant such as caffeine (found in tea or coffee), or a sedative, such as phenobarbitone, or an anti-sickness pill (an antiemetic), or several of these. In the United Kingdom simple analgesics can be bought by anyone in a chemist's shop. They are the mainstay of treatment of a migraine unless:

(1) you find you are taking too many in the course of a week. There are dangers of rebound headaches and other complications (discussed earlier) from taking too many, even simple, preparations

(2) you have difficulty in swallowing tablets in which case the effervescent forms of the same tablets can be taken or it becomes necessary to take ergot preparations which can be inhaled, sucked, chewed, used as suppositories or injected. Ergot preparations should only be obtained on a doctor's prescription

(3) an early symptom is vomiting, nausea or a stomach upset; or the tablets, even taken early at the beginning of an attack, are not readily absorbed. In this case various anti-sickness (antiemetic) tablets, prescribed by your doctor, can be taken before the analgesic to allay the sickness and settle the stomach.

A wide range of tablets can be prescribed by a doctor to reduce the number of migraine attacks and lessen their severity. It may still be necessary, particularly on starting prophylactic therapy, to take simple analgesics or antiemetics as described above. It does not help to take an extra prophylactic tablet at the time of an attack unless your doctor specifically advises you to do so, as most of these preventative tablets act too slowly to help an individual attack. Tablets can be equally effective in those migraine sufferers who have food and other allergies triggering off their attacks as in those who do not. Most antimigraine drugs can be taken in combination with other drugs, but if there is any question of doubt, especially if driving, check with your doctor.

NOTES ON THE MORE COMMONLY USED HEADACHE PREPARATIONS

This is not an inclusive list. Other varieties of drugs, including tranquillizers, anxietolytics and anticonvulsants may also be used.

Analgesics

(1) Single drugs
Aspirin: aspirins are available in many forms and, except in the presence of stomach or intestinal irritation and bleeding disorders, are usually

safe when properly used. Effervescent and soluble forms are most effective for migraine and headache. Dosage 300mg to 1000mg.

Paracetamol (Panadol): a safe derivative of phenacetin, but can be harmful in the presence of kidney disease. Compound drugs containing the parent substances — phenacetin — are best avoided. Paracetamol is available in effervescent form. Dosage 0.5 to 1gm.

Codeine: has a constipating effect and is less effective than either aspirin or paracetamol.

Fortral: pentozocine — rather slower acting than aspirin and paracetamol when taken by mouth, but effective as in injection.

Indocid — and many other analgesics — are primarily available for rheumatic disorders and tend to act too slowly to be effective for headaches.

(2) Compound preparations
(These are either combinations of analgesics or of analgesics plus antiemetics, sedatives or stimulants.)

Syndol: contains paracetamol, codeine, doxylamine and caffeine. A recently developed tablet with few side effects. Not recommended to children. Dosage 1–2 tablets every 4–6 hours.

Migraleve: the pink tablets contain buclizine,

paracetamol and codeine; the yellow tablets are similar but omit the antiemetic buclizine. Dosage 2 pink, followed if necessary by 2 yellow tablets two hours later, and the yellow tablets can be repeated every 4 hours.

Veganin: contains aspirin, paracetamol and codeine. Dosage 1–2 tablets every 4 hours.

Codis: contains aspirin and codeine. Dosage 1–2 tablets every 4 hours.

Fortagesic: contains pentazocine and paracetamol. Not recommended for children. Dosage 1–2 tablets every 4 hours.

Equagesic: contains ethoheptazine, meprobamate, aspirin and calcium carbonate. Not recommended for children. Dosage 2 tablets every 4 hours.

Ergot preparations

These have to be avoided in the presence of coronary heart disease, vascular disease, raised blood pressure, liver or kidney damage, sepsis, during pregnancy or with lactation. They are best avoided in children and in the treatment of complicated or focal migraine. There is a danger of chronic malaise from mild ergot overdosage, and more serious effects can follow sever intoxication.

Method of dosage	*Preparation*
Effervescent	*Effergot*: ergotamine tartrate 2mg, caffeine 50mg; ½–1 tablet dissolved in water at beginning of attack, followed by ½ tablet at 30 minute intervals. Maximum 3 daily or 5 in any week.
As a spray	*Medihaler-ergotamine* (metered dose aerosol): 1 dose, repeated if required after 5 minutes. Maximum 6 doses in 24 hours; 15 in any one week.
Under the tongue	*Lingraine*: ergotamine tartrate 2mg. 1 sublingually at onset of attack. If necessary, ½ tablet 1 hour later. Maximum 3 in 24 hours; 8 in any one week.
Chewed	*Cafergot Q*: ergotamine tartrate 1mg, caffeine 100 mg. 1–2 tablets at

	onset of attack. Maximum 4 daily; 10 in any one week.
Tablets, swallowed	*Dihydergot*: dihydroergotamine 1mg. 2–3 tablets repeated ½ hourly. Can be used 3 times daily prophylactically. Maximum 10 tablets in any one day. *Femergin*: ergotamine tartrate 1mg. 2–6 per attack. Maximum 6 daily; 10 in any one week. *Migril*: ergotamine tartrate 2mg, cyclizine, caffeine 1–2 tablets at onset of attack, ½–1 at 30 minute intervals. Maximum 4 daily; 6 in any one week.
Liquid form	*Dihydergot Oral Solution*: dihydroergotamine mesylate 2mg/ml. 20–30 drops repeated every 30 minutes as necessary. Maximum 100 drops daily.

Per rectum

Cafergot Suppositories: ergotamine tartrate 2mg, caffein, 100 mg, belladonna 0.25mg, butabital 100 mg. Avoid with glaucoma or prostatic enlargement. 1 at onset of attack or at night prophylactically. Maximum 3 daily; 5 in any one week.

By injection

Dihydergot: 1mg/ml 1–2mg subcutaneously or intramuscularly

Femergin: 0.5mg/ml. 0.25 mg to 0.5mg subcutaneously or intramuscularly.

Antiemetics (antisickness tablets)

Stemetil: prochlorperazine 5mg. May be used prophylactically, even for children. Adult dosage 1–3 tablets daily.

Torecan: thiethylperazine 10mg. 1–3 tablets daily. Not recommended for children. Can be given by injection.

Valoid: cyclizine 50mg. 1–3 tablets daily. Not for children under 10 years.

Mexalon: metoclopromide 10mg. 1–3 tablets daily. Can be given by injection. Not recommended for children.

Maxalon has the additional advantage in stimulating normal contraction of the stomach and intestine, thus overcoming a gastro-intestinal stasis.

Prophylactic drugs

Used to lessen frequency and severity of headaches. These drugs tend to act too slowly for treatment of any particular headache and ordinary analgesics may also be needed.

Dixarit: clonidine. Acts by stabilizing the tone of blood vessels. Although the mechanism is unknown, it appears to be particularly effective with migraine of dietary origin. Has few side effects but is used cautiously in people with low blood pressure. Dosage 0.025mg tablets, 2–6 daily.

Sanomigran: pizotifen 0.5mg. Related to methysergide but with fewer side effects. Reduces the uptake of noradrenaline and serotonin. Possesses sedative and antidepressant properties. Dosage 0.5mg, 3 times daily.

Deseril: methysergide 1mg. A powerful antimigraine drug which also has unfortunate side effects. However, it is safe when used for a limited number of weeks under medical control. Dosage 1mg 2–3 times daily.

Hormone therapy: bromocriptine, papaverine and reserpine have all been used experimentally. Hormone therapy is now established, but the particular preparation used depends upon expert advice.

Inderal: propranolol 40mg. A beta-blocker which maintains blood vessel tone and may also have a central action on the brain. Particularly helpful where migraine is accompanied by palpitations, but better avoided in allergic states and in those subject to heart failure. Dosage 40mg 3 times daily.

Arlington Pocket Guides
only £1.95 each

ABZ of Vitamins and Minerals
Earl Mindell

Anti-Acne Book
Dr David Murray

Pocket Guide to Contact Lenses
Nigel Burnett Hodd

Pocket Guide to Migraines and Headaches
Dr Edmund Critchley

Pocket Guide to Stress
Dr Dick Thompson

Where Do I Come From?
Claire Rayner

Available from your local bookshop. In case of difficulty, send a postal order or sterling cheque to Arlington Books at the address below (please add 50p for postage and packing):

Arlington Books (Publishers) Ltd
15–17 King Street, St James's, London SW1Y 6QU